FATTY LIVER DISEASE

DISCLAIMER

This book is not in any way a replacement of medical advice you may receive from any medical professional, such as a doctor or other healthcare provider. This book only contains general information about Fatty Liver Disease, including: types, causes, possible treatments, and suggested dietary plans.

This book strongly urges you to consult a doctor with any questions you may have, and encourages you to talk to a doctor about any information from this book that you feel is applicable to you. If you feel you may be suffering from any medical issues, seek help immediately. Never delay seeking medical advice, never disregard medical advice, or discontinue medical treatment because of information provided in this book.

This book is meant as an informative guide about Fatty Liver Disease. As with any condition you may have, it is important for you to do research on it, to get more of an understanding of what it is and what you can do for yourself. This book takes much of that research you would need to do and puts it into one guide for you, discussing the anatomy and function of the Liver, what Fatty Liver Disease is, the differences between Non-alocholic Fatty Liver Disease and Alocholic Fatty Liver Disease, and possible lifestyle changes you might need to do if you have Fatty Live Disease.

Once again, any information you learn from this book, you should consult with a doctor first before using.

Table Of Contents

Introduction: Fatty Liver Disease: What You Need To Know .. 4

Chapter One: Anatomy And Function Of The Liver 7

Chapter Two: What Is Fatty Liver? 11

Chapter Three: Types Of Fatty Liver 15

Chapter Four: Treatment, Risks, & Prevention 19

Chapter Five: What You Should Be Eating If You Have A Fatty Liver 26

Chapter Six: What You Shouldn't Be Eating If You Have A Fatty Liver 30

Chapter Seven: Dietary Plans For Fatty Liver 34

Chapter Eight: Diet Recipes For Fatty Liver 39

Chapter Nine: Home Remedies For Fatty Liver Disease 49

Chapter Ten: Final Message 52

INTRODUCTION
FATTY LIVER DISEASE: WHAT YOU NEED TO KNOW

The human body is a complicated network of parts that work together to keep us alive and healthy. We have the heart to pump blood throughout our bodies, we have the lungs to give us oxygen and get rid of carbon dioxide, and we have the brain to basically run the show. If someone were to mention "vital organs," these three would probably be the ones that popped into your head.

But really, these are just a few of the body's vital organs. Others often get overlooked. Of these overlooked organs, the liver is perhaps the most important. Its roles in our body are diverse, responsible for everything from the release of chemicals for digestion to the removal of toxins from our body. The body cannot live without the liver, and liver failure results in death without a liver transplant.

Because the liver is so important and once it has sustained a certain amount of damage, it requires a transplant, diseases of the liver are extremely serious. This book focuses on fatty liver disease, or FLD. Like any disease, especially when dealing with the liver, it's paramount to catch FLD before it becomes too serious to treat.

Because there are many different ways in which FLD can develop, it can affect a wide variety of people. Basically, everyone is at risk. The good news is that there are things you can do to avoid it, and even if you already have it, there are ways to treat it. It can take years for it to progress enough to require a transplant, so there is plenty of opportunity to discover it and change your lifestyle to ensure you live a long, healthy life.

If the direct cause of your FLD can be determined, it may be as simple as taking a few steps to reduce the build-up of fat. For example, if the cause is determined to be alcohol consumption, then it may be as easy as cutting down your consumption or avoiding alcohol completely.

However, if it is a more complicated issue, there may not be such a simple solution. It could be that you have diabetes and have developed FLD as a result. Diabetes can cause a number of issues in your body and you will need to carefully monitor your sugar intake and keep your blood sugar under control. If your FLD is a side-effect of obesity, you will most likely need to completely change your lifestyle, eating a healthy diet and exercising regularly in order to treat the condition.

Most people treat their bodies as "out of sight, out of mind," That is, if they don't go looking for something wrong, then there is nothing wrong. Even if people notice unusual symptoms, they often explain them away or ignore them until their condition becomes much worse and they have no choice but to see a medical professional. By no means are we suggesting that you should become a hypochondriac and rush to the doctor at the drop of a hat, but certainly take care of your body and see a doctor for any concerning symptoms.

With FLD, there really aren't any warning signs. It can only be diagnosed by a doctor with a blood test, which isn't included in routine bloodwork. If you are concerned that you might have FLD, it is best to discuss the possibility with your doctor and request the test.

That said, rather than waiting for something bad to happen, you can take steps now to try to avoid developing FLD at all. This book will educate you on what you can do to help yourself. Prevention is the best medicine, so even if you don't currently have FLD, steps taken in this book can reduce your risk of getting it and help you live a healthier life.

What it ultimately comes down to is treating your body right by eating well and getting plenty of exercise. It's okay to have fun and eat junk food once in a while or have a few drinks at the bar, but understand that those things are not only bad for you in general, but affect your liver, so they need to be done in moderation and balanced with a healthy, liver-friendly diet the rest of the time. This will ensure that your liver can function at optimum levels when you need it most.

CHAPTER ONE
ANATOMY AND FUNCTION OF THE LIVER

The liver is a vital organ in many animals, including humans. For humans, the liver is located in the abdomen, in the upper right quadrant, just below the diaphragm and above the stomach, gallbladder, pancreas, and the intestines.

The liver is the second largest organ in the body, weighing three pounds. (Fun fact: Our skin is our largest organ!) It is reddish-brown and shaped like a cone, consisting of two main sections called lobes, the left and right. If terminology like "lobe" reminds you of the brain, you won't be surprised to learn that just like the brain, the liver is highly complex.

The liver is a gland cited as having around 500 different functions. While we won't go over every function in this book, we will go over some of the most important ones. Generally, the liver is capable of breaking down complex molecules to help with digestion or to clear toxins from our bloodstream, amongst other things.

Because it plays such an important role in our bodies, it should be noted that there is currently no long-term solution for a failing liver, short of a liver transplant. There are short-term solutions, such as dialysis, which is basically when a patient is hooked up to a machine to detoxify the blood. It can help in some situations, but only for so long. Transplants are complicated and risky, not to mention difficult to come by, so the better option is to take care of your liver now to avoid needing a transplant in the future.

Main Functions Of The Liver

1. Secretion Of Bile

Bile is a yellowish-brown to dark green substance that is constantly produced by our livers and stored in our gallbladders. Its primary purpose is to help break down fats when digesting food to make it easier for the stomach to digest, but it also prevents fats from reforming into complex fats. Bile can also help extract bilirium, which is formed from hemoglobin and glucuronidation as a result of the liver recycling red blood cells.

2. Blood Purification

The liver contains special cells called Kupffer cells, which are responsible for the capture and digestion of:

- Bacteria
- Fungi
- Parasites
- Viruses
- Drugs
- Food additives
- Alcohol
- Pesticides
- and other foreign material (that doesn't belong in the body).

3. Storing Glucose

When food is digested, the liver takes carbohydrates and basically converts it into glucose. Glucose acts as a fuel for the body. The liver doesn't release all of the glucose it produces, and will take a portion of the glucose and transform it into glycogen. If the glucose levels in the body are low, the liver will transform the glycogen back into glucose.

4. Lipid (Fat) Metabolism

Another function of the liver is the breakdown of fats, also known as lipids. It can create many things useful for the body, including Adenosine Triphosphate (ATP), cholesterol, and lipoproteins.

ATP is used to carry energy in and out of cells for any number of things, including the synthesis of proteins and cell membranes, help with cell movement, and cell division.

Cholesterol is a term you've probably heard before, but you most likely think of it as something bad or something to avoid. The truth is that cholesterol is not bad in most cases. For example, the liver produces cholesterol to help with the production of bile, give cells a cell wall, and produce some of the body's hormones.

Lipoproteins are a way of transporting fatty acids through the bloodstream to wherever they are needed, including the cells and liver.

5. Protein Metabolism

When protein goes through digestion, it is broken down into amino acids. The liver then uses amino acids to create other things it needs, but before doing so, must remove the amine group from the structures. The amine group is then transformed into urea and ammonia, which are waste products are are secreted, usually through urine. The liver then uses the remaining amino acids to produce different kinds or proteins, including those that help with clotting, and ATP.

6. Storage

The Liver acts as a storage container for many chemicals, and then releases them as needed. Some are produced by the liver, such as glucose, and others are absorbed by the liver, such as iron and copper from red blood cells. The liver also stores Vitamins A, D, E, K, and B12.

7. Fetal Blood Supply

The liver in a fetus is not used for its normal digestive functions because a fetus does not really digest food, but gets nutrition from the placenta. Instead, the liver is responsible for creating blood stem cells for the fetus. After birth, this function is given to red bone marrow, and the liver begins its digestive functions.

As you can see, even from this short list, the liver's functions in the body are very diverse. We mentioned only 7 out of 500 functions! Knowing that the liver is such an important organ with hundreds of functions, you should be inspired to do what you can to treat your Liver well. The harsh truth is that if you don't, you could die. For a long a happy life, treat your liver right.

CHAPTER TWO
WHAT IS FATTY LIVER?

Fatty liver disease is the build-up of a special fat called triglyceride, which is composed of glycerol and three fatty acids. This build-up in the liver is called hepatic steatosis. Hepat is the Greek word for liver, and steatosis refers to fat build-up in cells (not just the liver). Throughout this book, you will see many words begin hepat-, such as hepatitis, in relation to the liver.

It is completely normal to have fat in most areas of your body, including your liver. With the liver, about five to ten percent fat is normal. The problem develops when fat builds up above normal levels. There are a host of things that can cause fat to build up in your body, and when fat builds up in the liver, it causes FLD.

Fortunately, is most cases, FLD is a reversible condition that can be resolved with lifestyle changes. If you drink too much, drink less. If you eat fast food every day, eat a healthier diet. It can be as simple as that, but it requires a lifetime commitment, and is not something you can do on a whim, or do just enough to get healthy and then go back to your old habits.

The difficulty with FLD is that it often doesn't cause unique symptoms, and most people don't know they have it. This is because the liver constantly works to repair itself from the damage that we do it. Early on in life, this is an easy task for the liver, but as one gets older, this may cause permanent scarring, which is what we call cirrhosis. Cirrhosis only occurs in the most extreme cases, such as overeating in the case of obesity, or binge-drinking with alcoholics.

A good reason to read this book and educate yourself on FLD is how common it is. FLD affects upwards of 30% of Americans (roughly 90 million people), while other countries around the world only see 10% - 25% of their populations affected. Meaning that if you're an American, you have great chance than people of other nationalities. Especially if you have an unhealthy lifestyle, you should consider the possibility that you might have or develop FLD, Either way, it is a good idea to get checked out by a doctor. Better to find it early than wait so long that it's too late to do anything.

More often than not, FLD is found in people over the age of 40, as it generally culminates over a lifetime, but it's not unheard of for children to have FLD. Don't let your age stop you from getting checked or considering a healthier lifestyle, because when FLD occurs and is untreated, it can lead to complications and even death.

Symptoms

There are no definitive signs of FLD, and the symptoms that are associated with it could also be the result of another condition. Generally, FLD is discovered as a result of another condition that may or may not be related to it, as FLD can cause a host of complications. For this reason, the discovery of FLD generally occurs when doctors are looking for something else.

There are some symptoms that could indicate a problem with your liver, potentially FLD:

- Constantly feeling tired or worn out
- Rapid weight loss
- Loss of appetite
- Nausea
- Non-specific abdominal pain
- Difficulty concentrating
- Yellowing of skin

The problem is, many of those symptoms could also describe someone with the flu or even AIDS. If you experience any of these symptoms, your best bet is to visit your doctor, who can help you determine the cause.

For FLD, a doctor will notice liver enzymes in your blood or an increase of iron. From there, your doctor may order an ultrasound and/or an MRI. With an MRI, a doctor can see how big your liver is, but that isn't definitive proof that something is wrong. Your doctor will likely ask about your consumption of alcohol, which could be a factor of FLD. Generally, less than two alcoholic drinks per day indicates non-alcoholic fatty liver disease (NAFLD), whereas two or more indicates alcoholic fatty liver, the first stage of alcoholic liver disease.

If a doctor believes that you do have FLD, they will do a liver biopsy. This will most likely be done at a clinic or a hospital, so they can provide you an anesthetic. This procedure involves inserting a needle in your abdomen to remove tissue from your liver for further examination, which will definitively tell them if you suffer from FLD, and the exact cause.

Causes

There are quite a number of things that cause fat build-up in your liver, but the causes are generally divided into five categories:

- **Metabolic** (primarily in the processing of fats in your system)
- **Nutritional** (whether you are getting the nutrients your body needs)
- **Drugs** (a number of drugs can cause the development of FLD)
- **Alcohol** (consumption of alcohol is one of the leading causes of FLD)
- **Other** (diseases with FLD as a side effect, etc.)

The exhaustive list of what can cause FLD contains too many to include here, but in this book will go over some of the most common ones. Of course, your doctor can give you more in-depth information about the various causes of FLD. A few of them are:

- **Malnutrition**
- **Severe Weight Loss**
- **Drugs** (such as amiodarone or methotrexate)
- **Alcohol**
- **Celiac Disease**
- **HIV**

Hepatitis C

CHAPTER THREE
TYPES OF FATTY LIVER

While this could have been included in Chapter Two, the importance of knowing the different types of fatty liver disease necessitates that we give the subject its own chapter. Understanding the different types of FLD will help guide you in what lifestyle changes you might make and how serious your condition may be.

Non-Alcoholic Fatty Liver Disease

Non-alcoholic fatty liver disease (NAFLD) is vague term used to describe the various reasons a liver might start accumulating fat besides alcohol consumption. Unlike NASH (listed below), this is only the presence of excess fat in the liver, greater than 10% of the liver's weight.

NAFLD is the most common form of FLD. Although anyone can get it, it is most common in people over 40 who are at risk for heart disease, are obese, or have diabetes. Generally, the fat has accumulated over many years, but can also be the result of childhood obesity.

Whatever the cause is determined to be, it is very treatable. The next chapter will talk about ways you can prevent and treat NAFLD.

Alcoholic Fatty Liver Disease

Alcoholic liver disease (ALD) begins with alcohol-induced fatty liver disease, and refers specifically to FLD that is brought on by excessive drinking. The liver considers alcohol to be a toxin, and will try to rid your body of it. However, the liver damages itself in the process. The occasional drink won't hurt you and your liver will recover. Heavy drinking, however, is a much different story.

It's best to note what is considered light drinking versus heavy drinking. While every person is different, and it is always best to consult your doctor about what is best for you specifically, it's generally accepted to be light drinking if you have only one drink a day and heavy drinking if you have two or more. Men with larger bodies might be able to have two drinks a day while remaining healthy.

This raises another question: What is it actually meant by the term "drink?" Generally, a drink is considered:

- A 12-ounce bottle of beer (5% alcohol)
- A 5-ounce glass of wine (12% alcohol)
- 1 ounce of spirits or hard liquor (40% alcohol)

Most people develop ALD after a short period of heavy drinking. The longer the drinking continues, the worse it gets. Fortunately, at the fattly liver stage, it is quite treatable. Either reduce your alcohol consumption or stop drinking entirely. If you have a large amount of alcohol in a short period, give your body a few weeks to recover before drinking again, as even a weekend of binge-drinking can give you ALD. If left untreated, ALD can lead to alcoholic hepatitis.

Non-Alcoholic Steatohepatitis (NASH)

If left untreated, NAFLD can lead to non-alcoholic steatohepatitis (NASH). You'll see the word "hepatitis" in there, which describes an inflammation of the liver. NASH is categorized by an excessive amount of fat in the liver, inflammation, and scarring. All of this can lead to cirrhosis (irreversible scarring/damage to the liver) and liver failure. It is estimated that 5% (15 million) of the US population has NASH.

It can take a number of years for NAFLD to become NASH, so if you go to a doctor for regular checkups, be sure they are checking the liver enzymes in your blood. If you have NASH, and it is caught early enough, a lifestyle change can reverse the effects. However, if you are suffering from cirrhosis, your options are quite limited. At the time of writing, there is no medical option to permanently stop or reverse cirrhosis, short of a liver transplant. That may change in the future with newly developed medication, so be sure to consult a doctor about your options if you have NASH.

Alcoholic Hepatitis

Alcoholic hepatitis is seen in heavy drinkers that drink heavily over an extended period of time, generally years. Like NASH, this is seen as increased fat in the Liver and inflammation. It's believed that 35% of heavy drinkers develop alcoholic hepatitis, especially if they are untreated alcoholics.

Alcoholic hepatitis can be mild or severe.

Mild alcoholic hepatitis can last for several years and will continuously damage the liver. The mild form is reversible if the sufferer stops drinking, but it can take several years to undo the damage. It is also likely that the person would never be able to drink again in their lives.

Severe alcoholic hepatitis may occur after someone with ALD binge-drinks, which causes alcoholic cirrhosis. Alcoholic cirrhosis is considered the third stage of ALD, and refers to irreversible scarring of the Liver. Cirrhosis may also develop from mild alcoholic hepatitis if the individual continues to drink, even lightly, for more than ten years.

Alcoholic cirrhosis is a life threatening condition. It is estimated that 10 - 15% of heavy drinkers develop alcholic cirrhosis.

Acute Fatty Liver Of Pregnancy

While rare, it is possible for FLD to develop during the third trimester of pregnancy. It can also occur after delivery. Symptoms may include nausea, vomiting, lack of appetite, and abdominal pain. Some symptoms can be confused with normal pregnancy symptoms, but about 70% of women diagnosed report yellowing of the skin and a high fever.

It was once believed that this was fatal to all pregnant women, but it is now treatable. It is still very serious, and once the liver is stabilized, doctors may make plans to induce early labor or perform a Cesarean section (C-Section).

CHAPTER FOUR
TREATMENT, RISKS, & PREVENTION

Fatty liver disease is relatively unknown when it comes to what average people know about their health. In fact, most people don't give much thought to their liver unless something is wrong. Even the media ignores liver diseases in favor of heart disease and cancer. FLD is a major problem that needs to be discussed.

In this section, we'll go over the treatments, risks, and preventative measures you can take when it comes to FLD. You will notice that treatment and prevention are primarily eating right and getting plenty of exercise, which are things you should do anyway to live a healthy life.

Treatment

Treatment of FLD often involves a lifestyle change. The cause of your FLD will determine what you need to do in your life to reduce the fat build-up. Generally, this includes one (or more) of the following:

- Reduction (or elimination) of alcohol consumption
- Losing weight
- Keeping your cholesterol down
- Managing your blood sugar

Things like high cholesterol or diabetes may be helped by medication, but being a heavy drinker or overweight will require you to change your lifestyle. Losing weight is an especially difficult lifestyle change, as you will need to completely revamp your diet and commit to exercising regularly.

Eating the right kinds of food can not only help you be healthier, but also help you reduce fat in your liver. More than eating the right kinds of foods, there are things you need to avoid, such as alcohol and fatty foods, which tend to be high in sugar. Generally, you want a lot of fresh fruits, vegetables, and whole grains, with a good source of lean protein.

However, if the problem becomes more serious, there are treatment options to consider. Every day there are new drugs treating diseases in new ways. By the time you read this, there may be something new on the market, so always consult your doctor with any questions you have. Generally, anything that can help you lower your cholesterol and manage your blood sugar will help with FLD in the long run.

There are many products on the market you can take, such as supplements. Remember that not all supplements have, or require, FDA approval. Some supplements have shown promise, such as Berberine and Vitamin D3. Some studies have been conducted on both in relation to FLD, with Berberine able to lower cholesterol, and D3 able to increase the amount of vitamin D in an NAFLD patient's body, since they are at risk of being vitamin D-deficient.

Risks

Before we can talk about prevention, we must first understand who is at risk for FLD. The simple answer is everyone, as anyone can develop this, but it is better if we explore this in more depth, as some are more at risk than others.

Factors that can contribute to FLD:

- Obesity
- Diabetes
- Alcohol consumption
- Drug abuse
- Pregnancy
- Malnutrition
- High blood pressure
- Genetic predisposition (common in your family)
- Rapid weight loss
- Hepatitis C

When it comes to NAFLD, those who are overweight are the most at risk. When you have a lot of excess weight on your body, known as obesity, you may have visceral fat developing. Visceral fat is fat that is sandwiched between your organs and your outer-body fat. Visceral fat can cause inflammation of the liver, which can cause liver damage.

However, do not assume that only those who are obese are at risk for NAFLD. In fact, even those who are lean/slender can be at risk. Most surprising is that studies have shown that while they do not show any of the classic signs an obese person does when developing NAFLD, lean people are twelve times more likely to die from NAFLD than obese individuals.

The most common reason lean people develop NAFLD is genetic predisposition to it. One genetic abnormality that increases your risk of NAFLD is a lisosomal acid lipase deficiency, which lowers the level of the enzyme that helps break down fats in our bodies, and causes the liver to accumulate it. Only about 16% of cases of NAFLD are lean, non-diabetic individuals, so it is rather uncommon.

Stress seems to be another factor in the development of NAFLD. Stress can do interesting things to our bodies, including causing weight loss and loss of appetite. Studies have shown in mice that stress can cause inflammation of the liver, reduce the amount of fat being processed, and cause NAFLD.

Preventions

Most people only start to be concerned about their liver once there is a problem. That is the wrong way to think about your liver, or even just your body in general. The best way to prevent problems with your body, whether it be diabetes, obesity, or even FLD, is to live a healthy lifestyle.

Now, no one is saying you can't enjoy a triple bacon cheeseburger or go out drinking with your friends. We are simply saying that it cannot be a normal diet for you. Eating like this once in a while is fine, but continuously doing so can have great consequences, such as developing FLD. The next two chapters will go over what you should and should not eat with FLD/what you should eat and not eat to prevent the development of FLD.

With alcohol consumption, it's important to give your body a break from alcohol in order to recover. Think of it as running a marathon. You run 26 miles. You're tired and exhausted. Now the last thing you want to do is to run another mile, much less another marathon. You want to rest and recover. This is what is going on for your liver. You consume a large amount of alcohol on Friday night and your liver is working overtime to remove that toxin from your system. Saturday comes, and you're out again, drinking the night away. Your liver can't keep up.

Below are a few additional things to consider when it comes to making changes to your lifestyle. As stated many times throughout this book, these changes will not only help prevent FLD, but improve your health overall.

1. **Eliminate high fructose corn syrup (HFCS).** HFCS is made from corn starch, and is found in a lot of processed foods as a food preservative, but also as a replacement for sugar. While there is a lot of conflicting studies and scientists are confused about why it is bad, many do agree that large consumption of any sweetener is bad. Given that HFCS has two types of sugars in it, it is best to avoid it.

2. **Eliminate white, processed flour.** Processed foods are generally bad, but this is especially true in the case of flour, as it means that the fiber is stripped away. Processed flour also represents what we call bad carbohydrates that, when consumed, can easily turn into sugar. It is better to eat whole grains and avoid any processed flours.

3. **Eat healthy fats.** We are often taught that we should avoid fats in our diet as much as possible. However, some fats are actually good for us. Healthy fats, also known as monounsaturated fats can increase our high-density lipoprotein (HDL, good fats), and lower our low-density

lipoprotein (LDL, bad fats). We will discuss some good sources of fats in the coming chapters.

4. **Exercise.** Exercise is important for a number of reasons, but in this case, especially because it can help manage insulin in your body (which help with your body digesting sugar), as well as reduce fat in your body, especially your liver. Even a simple 30-minute walk can do wonders for your body in preventing FLD.

5. **Eat detoxifying foods.** Foods like broccoli, cauliflower, Burssels' sprouts, kale, collards, cabbage, arugula, and watercress can help detoxify your body and in some ways help repair your liver.

6. **Be careful of the protein you eat.** Meat is a good source of protein, but not all meats are good for you. Consider consuming lean meats such as chicken and fish or lean read meat. You have other protein options, as well, which will be discussed in the coming chapters. Try to have a protein with every meal, whatever it be.

7. **Consume as much Omega-3 as you can.** Omega-3 is a fatty acid that has many health benefits. Studies have shown that those low in Omega-3 have a higher risk of developing FLD. We will discuss good sources of Omega-3 in the coming chapters.

8. **Drink coffee.** A few cups of coffee and tea have been shown to reduce FLD in mice with a high-fat diet. It is believed that the caffeine is the reason why, though the extra sugar people add can cause problems for your liver, so try to cut back on that. Soda drinkers, try real sugar

alternatives or cutting soda from your diet if you're feeling strong.

9. **Eat lots of fiber.** As we all know, fiber often increases the frequency with which we use the restroom, but this is a good thing! It detoxifies your body. Oftentimes, toxins can build up in your body and fiber can help eliminate that, assisting your liver.

Once again, this is a list of things you should do to prevent FLD. The rest of this book will be focused on what to do if you already have FLD. In our next chapter, we will discuss what you should eat if you have FLD, and the following chapter will describe what you shouldn't eat. You will no doubt notice that much of what we've listed in the prevention section is very similar to the information presented in the next two chapters, so you can read the next two chapters as an extension of ways to prevent FLD.

CHAPTER FIVE
WHAT YOU SHOULD BE EATING IF YOU HAVE A FATTY LIVER

In the last section, we discussed what foods you should and shouldn't eat to prevent the development of fatty liver disease, but in this section we'll talk more about what you should eat if you already have FLD. Remember, treating FLD means changing your lifestyle, so don't expect it to be as simple as eating a few vegetables and calling it a day.

When eating with non-alcoholic fatty liver disease, the goal to accomplish a few specific things:

- Reduce fat in the liver
- Help the liver repair itself
- Induce production of insulin
- Lose weight

The suggestions in this book are by no means an official diet plan for those suffering from NAFLD, but rather some guidelines to consider or speak with your doctor about, as you may have additional concerns in relation to your health that may affect what you eat and your portion sizes.

When most people hear the word diet, they think of eating less. The advice you will receive in this book is that you should satisfy your hunger needs. You're hungry for a reason. If you need a lot of food, you should eat a lot of food, especially if you do a high-energy workout work in a labor-intensive occupation. The most important thing is that you are eating the right kinds of foods.

Fruits And Vegetables

All your life, you've heard that you should eat your vegetables. Well, you should. Both fruits and vegetables provide an array of nutrients, including vitamins, minerals, and antioxidants. Fruits and vegetables help strengthen your body's immune system, which helps in dealing with infections and diseases. The American Liver Foundation also recommends a diet rich in fruits and vegetables to help reduce symptoms of FLD.

Fruits and vegetables are both low in calories, which makes them great foods to have in addition to of other foods as a meal, or alone as a snack. Fruits, however, do tend to be fairly high in sugar, so you'll need to limit yourself to two pieces of fruit a day. You can basically eat as many vegetables as you like.

You can eat basically any fruits and vegetables you like, but these are particularly high in antioxidants: blueberries, cherries, raspberries, oranges, grapefruit, papaya, tomatoes, spinach, broccoli, kale, mustard greens, and bell peppers.

Proteins

You can get protein from a variety of sources, mostly from meats and nuts, but also from a few vegetables. The most important thing to consider when you are choosing meats to eat when you have FLD is what the animal ate. Animals that were fed plants such as grass or algae tend to be ideal.

You should avoid any meat that is grain-fed. Grain is often given to animals, such as cows, as a cheap way to fatten them up. This is why grass-fed only animals are more expensive.

Fish is an ideal choice, either canned or fresh. Poultry is also a good choice, but you should try to go for lean, white meat over the fatty, dark meat. You can also consume grass-fed lean red meat.

If you would like another option, eggs are a good source of protein, but the yolk is high in fat, so you should really only eat the whites. If you like the flavor of the yolk, it's fine to eat, as long as you remember to do so in moderation.

Don't forget that you can also get protein from nuts and legumes, like beans, chickpeas, and lentils.

Be wary of protein powders. Double check what a powder contains before buying it. You want to avoid sugar as much as possible. Check that the protein powder you're considering doesn't contain sugar. Look for powders that contain stevia, a natural sweetener.

Whole Grains

As mentioned in Chapter Four, there is a concern when it comes to grains, as they contain carbohydrates. There are both good carbs and bad carbs. Whole grains are good carbs. Whole grains have vitamins, minerals, antioxidants, and dietary fiber, which are missing in processed grains. They are low-glycemic, which means they do not contain a lot of sugar.

A diet that includes whole grains can help reduce heart disease, diabetes, and FLD. It is also a good food to eat to encourage the liver to repair itself. Foods that are high in whole grains are: oats, bulgur, spelt, barley, brown or wild rice, and rye. Many of these will also make you feel more full after eating them, which can be good for weight loss, as you will have less desire to overeat.

Unsaturated Fats

Fat is an ugly word in the world of dieting. We tend to believe that all fats are bad, but that's simply not true. Unsaturated fats are quite healthy for us. It's the saturated and trans fats that we should avoid. What makes unsaturated fats so great is that they help with heart health, brain function, and overall physical wellness. They also help the body absorb nutrients from other foods, so it is an especially good idea to combine these fats with vegetables. Some sources of unsaturated fats are olive oil, canola oil, walnuts, almonds, avocados, and seeds.

One type of unsaturated fat, is called monounsaturated fat, otherwise known as Omega-3. A good source of Omega-3s are fish, such as salmon, tuna, mackerel, and sardines. They can also be found in walnuts and canola oil.

Now that we have an idea of all the things we can and should eat, we can focus on what we shouldn't eat.

CHAPTER SIX
WHAT YOU SHOULDN'T BE EATING IF YOU HAVE A FATTY LIVER

We've discussed what you should be eating if you have Fatty Liver Disease. Now, we'll talk about what you should avoid.

If you develop Non-Alcoholic Fatty Liver Disease, then it should be rather easy for you to identify the foods that you should avoid, as there is a good chance, especially if you're obese, that these are the foods you already consume. Even if you're not obese, and simply a victim of genetics, this section will still be of benefit to you.

I will stress that if you're diagnosed with NAFLD, changing your diet is crucial, and knowing what foods to avoid is paramount. Only through a proper diet can one hope to avoid a more serious condition such as cirrhosis and liver failure. Most doctors should agree with what is featured in this section, but still consult with your doctor after reading to figure out what is best for you.

Fast Food

It should come as no surprise that fast food is unhealthy for you. While many fast food joints are beginning to offer healthier options on their menus, the healthiest choice of all is to stay away from fast food entirely. Many places make use of deep-frying, which means their food is full of saturated fats. These places also serve processed foods that have lost most of their nutritional value during processing. If that wasn't enough, it is likely that sugar or high fructose corn syrup is added to make the food taste sweeter.

All of this is just plain bad for a healthy diet, and there is very little health benefit gained from fast food. Fast food should be avoided at all costs when you have FLD, even as a once-in-awhile guilty pleasure. Instead, make food from home, and even if friends and coworkers want to go to a Fast Food join, bring your food with you.

Junk Food

Junk food is another thing to avoid, and is on par with fast food. Junk food is a term used to describe anything from a bag of chips or a candy bar. Typically, junk foods use high fructose corn syrup as a preservative and sweetener, although some companies have tried switching to healthier alternatives. Some soda companies use real sugar and some potato chip companies use unsaturated fats, but these products still tend to be full of fat and low in nutritional value.

Like fast food, it is best to avoid junk food is you have NAFLD. You might not think they taste as good, but fresh raw vegetables make a much better snack than a bag of chips.

Processed Grains

Processed grains tend to have many of their nutrients removed during processing, including fiber. These processed grains are also full of carbohydrates, or carbs, which become sugar when we digest them, and affect our blood sugar level, which is bad for our liver. Because processed grains are more easily digested, we often become hungry quickly, and feel the need to eat more. Whole grains make us feel more full when we eat, give us energy throughout the day, and keep us from eating more than we need to.

Alcohol

Obviously, alcohol consumption contributes to the development of alcoholic fatty liver disease, and it should similarly be avoided for those with NAFLD. This is because alcohol can exasperate and damage a fatty liver, but also because alcohol can be converted to sugar in our bodies and affect our blood sugar levels. While small amounts aren't going to hurt you, they don't do you any good, either. You should reduce your alcohol consumption or stop drinking when you have NAFLD.

Other Foods To Avoid

There no possible way to cover every food you should avoid and the specific reasons why in this space. Here is a general list of other foods we haven't covered that aren't good for you. Some of the foods on the list may be things you can consume in smaller quantities, while others are things to avoid completely. Generally, avoiding all of these is a safe bet, but you can do further research and consult with your doctor if you do not wish to avoid one or more of the foods on the list.

- Dairy products
- Watermelon
- Raisins
- Bananas

- Corn and corn-based products
- Chocolate
- Candy
- "Diet" anything
- Pizza
- White Rice
- Mangos
- Grapes
- Butter and margarine
- Fried anything

In the last two chapters, we've listed what you should and should not eat when you have FLD, specifically NAFLD. We've covered a lot of information in a short amount of time, so don't feel bad if you feel a little overwhelmed. The next few sections will help you create a plan for yourself that keeps what you've learned so far in mind.

CHAPTER SEVEN
DIETARY PLANS FOR FATTY LIVER

When it comes to changing your lifestyle, it's not enough to just have the right foods, you must reorganize your life around proper eating. You shouldn't treat it as getting healthy enough to go back to your old ways, but rather a lifetime commitment to eating right to stay healthy for as long as you can.

While the next few sections are dedicated to food, it is still important to note that healthy eating means nothing unless you are also exercising. Be sure to get out there and work those calories off.

In this section, we'll go over some plans for you to consider when you have Fatty Liver Disease.

Good Foods For Fatty Liver

Oats

Oatmeal is your friend. Get a bowl of oatmeal and add in some dry fruits, walnuts, or even honey to improve the taste and make your meal even more healthy. This will lower your blood sugar and improve digestion. Also make sure you eat a good portion of this, as it will give you a boost of energy that lasts several hours.

Dairy

While you should avoid most dairy, such as cheese that is high in fat, there are some dairy items that you can have as a snack or a replacement for breakfast. Good foods are: yogurt, buttermilk, cottage cheese, and kefir. This will improve digestion and remove fats from your body.

Fruits and Vegetables

Fruits and vegetables are a great way to get a lot of vitamins and minerals. While you do want to limit your fruit, as it can be high in sugar, you can enjoy vegetables as much as you want, either as a snack or with other things we eat.

Light Days

Throughout the week, have a few days where you eat like a vegetarian. Eat vegetables, whole grains, beans, and nuts. Many of these are foods of which you can have as much as you want, so don't be afraid to eat until full. This will give your liver a break.

Water

We haven't really talked about water in this book, but water is absolutely necessary for you. You must drink quite a bit of water throughout the day. Generally 64 ounces, but don't worry if you don't hit that number, as long as you are trying to drink a lot of water. Most waters should be OK, but do avoid any water that have added ingredients.

Many believe that flavored sports drinks are a replacement for water. They are only ideal for high-energy workouts where you lose a lot of sweat and are active for several hours. Even if you work out, water should usually be all you need.

You can add some fruits or vegetables to your water for taste, like berries, cucumber, or lemon.

Meal Frequency

While you should eat until you feel satisfied, it is actually better to eat smaller meals throughout the day. It is recommended to have five meals in a day, with two larger meals such as breakfast and dinner, and a series of smaller meals that are more like snacks.

You could also have three larger meals, with snacks throughout the day if you want. Change this to what will work best for you, but instead of eating everything in just three meals, you should divide it up throughout the day. The benefit of doing this is that it will leave you feeling satisfied and energized throughout the day, and will be easier on your liver.

Weekly Meal Plan For Fatty Liver

Below is a suggested meal plan with foods you could eat throughout the week. This is by no means exactly what you should do, and you should adapt this to your specific needs and even to what you prefer to eat, within the guidelines mentioned in this book and after consulting a medcal professional.

This section is simply to give you an idea of what you could do.

Monday

Breakfast: Oatmeal with blueberries

Snacks: 1/4 cup of nuts
Lunch: Salad
Snacks: One carrot
Dinner: Brown rice with grilled turkey breasts

Tuesday

Breakfast: Guacamole on two pieces of toast
Snacks: Two medium-sized apples
Lunch: Vegetable soup and quinoa with beans
Snacks: One cup of low fat yogurt
Dinner: Barley-stuffed poblanos

Wednesday

Breakfast: Chia pudding with berries and half a tbsp of honey
Snacks: A cup of homemade popcorn (use no oil/butter!)
Lunch: One eggplant boat
Snacks: A bowl of fresh fruit
Dinner: Cilantro lime grilled tofu skewers

Thursday

Breakfast: Egg-white omelette
Snacks: One Chia Bar
Lunch: Lentil salad with eggs
Snacks: Vegetable smoothie
Dinner: Big slice of grilled or oven-baked salmon with leafy greens salad

Friday

Breakfast: Yogurt
Snacks: Mixed vegetables
Lunch: Lean chicken wrap
Snacks: Handful of nuts
Dinner: Large salad

Saturday

Breakfast: Bowl of fruit
Snacks: Graham crackers
Lunch: Vegetable soup and tuna wrap
Snacks: Yogurt
Dinner: Three bean and kale salad

Sunday

Breakfast: Cottage cheese on two slices of toast
Snacks: Two apples
Lunch: Vegetable soup
Snacks: Boiled cauliflower puree
Dinner: Green beans with roasted onions

CHAPTER EIGHT
DIET RECIPES FOR FATTY LIVER

Vegan Cauliflower Wings

Total time: 1 hour
Prep time: 10 minutes
Cook time: 50 minutes
Serves: 2-4

Ingredients

Wings

1 large head of cauliflower cut into florets
1/2 cup unsweetened almond milk
1/2 cup water
3/4 cup all-purpose or rice flour
2 tsp garlic powder
2 tsp onion powder
1 tsp cumin
1 tsp paprika
1/4 tsp sea salt
1/4 tsp ground pepper

BBQ Sauce
1 tbsp vegan butter, melted
Your favorite bottled sauce (try to pick something with low sugar)

Salt & Vinegar Sauce

1 tbsp vegan butter, melted
3 tbsp apple cider vinegar
1 tbsp water
Sea salt, to taste

Directions

Preheat oven to 450 degrees.

Line two baking sheets with parchment paper.

Mix all wing ingredients (besides cauliflower) in a large mixing bowl. Submerge each cauliflower floret into the mix and tap off the excess on the side of the bowl. Place the dipped florets in a single layer on the prepared baking sheets.

Bake 15 minutes then flip to brown on the other side. Bake another 10 minutes or until golden brown. Remember to use gloves or towel when handling hot surfaces inside the oven!

While baking, prepare the sauce of your choice (or both) in a large bowl (or two).

Remove the cauliflower from the oven, put the florets into the sauce(s), and toss to coat. Place the florets back onto the baking sheets in a single layer. If you are using the Salt & Vinegar sauce, sprinkle the cauliflower florets with sea salt.

Bake another 25 minutes – flipping the florets over halfway through the bake time.

If you have any sauce leftover, brush it onto the cauliflower florets after removing them from the oven.

You can serve the BBQ wings with with your favorite Ranch dressing.

Portobello "Philly Cheese Steak"

Total time: 20 minutes
Prep time: 5 minutes
Cook time: 15 minutes
Serves: 4

Ingredients

2 tsp extra-virgin olive oil
1 medium onion, sliced
4 large portobello mushrooms, stems and gills removed, sliced
1 large red bell pepper, thinly sliced
2 tsp dried oregano
1/2 tsp freshly ground pepper
1 tbsp all-purpose flour
1/4 cup vegetable broth
1 tbsp reduced-sodium soy sauce
3 oz thinly sliced reduced-fat provolone cheese or vegan cheese
4 whole-wheat rolls, split and toasted

Directions

Heat oil in a large nonstick skillet over medium-high heat. Add onion and cook, stirring often, until soft and beginning to brown, for about 5 minutes. Add mushrooms, bell pepper, oregano, and pepper. Cook, stirring often, until the vegetables are wilted and soft, about 7 minutes.

Reduce heat to low. Sprinkle the vegetables with flour and stir to coat. Stir in broth and soy sauce. Bring to a simmer.

Remove from heat, lay cheese slices on top of the vegetables, cover, and let stand until melted, 1 to 2 minutes.

Divide the mixture into 4 portions with a spatula, leaving the melted cheese layer on top. Scoop a portion onto each toasted bun and serve immediately.

Roasted Bok Choy

Total time: 17 minutes
Prep time: 2 minutes
Cook time: 15 minutes
Servings: 4-6

Ingredients

6 heads of baby bokchoy
Olive oil (or oil of your liking)
Salt and pepper, to taste

Directions

Preheat oven to 450 degrees.

Cut each bokchoy head in half lengthwise and place on baking sheet. Lightly drizzle with oil, sprinkle with salt and pepper, and toss to coat.

Roast the bokchoy cut side down for 10 minutes. After 10 minutes flip each bokchoy over and roast for another 5 minutes.

Serve as a side with chicken or pork.

Liver-Friendly Tacos – Quinoa Taco Meat

Total time: 1 hour
Prep time: 15 minutes
Cook time: 30 minutes

Ingredients

Quinoa

1 cup rinsed tri-color, white, or red quinoa
1 cup vegetable broth
3/4 cup water

Seasonings

1/2 cup of your favorite salsa
1 tbsp nutritional yeast
2 tsp ground cumin
2 tsp ground chili powder
1/2 tsp garlic powder
1/2 tsp each sea salt and black pepper
1 tbsp olive or avocado oil

Directions

Put quinoa into a medium saucepan with vegetable broth and water and bring to a boil. Then reduce heat, cover, and let simmer for 15 to 20 minutes, or until the liquid has been absorbed.

Add in the remaining ingredients and stir thoroughly. Let cook for an additional 10 minutes on low heat, stirring occasionally.

Use a whole grain tortilla and mixture to create a burrito or a taco. Top with additional salsa, if desired.

Healthy Black Bean Brownies

Total time: 30 minutes
Prep time: 2 minutes
Cook time: 18 minutes
Serves: 9-12

Ingredients

1 15-oz can organic black beans, drained and rinsed very well
2 tbsp cocoa powder
1/2 cup quick oats
1/4 tsp salt
1/2 cup pure maple syrup
1/4 cup coconut oil
2 tsp alcohol-free pure vanilla extract
1/2 tsp baking powder
1/2 cup chocolate chips

Directions

Preheat oven to 350 degrees.

Combine all ingredients except chocolate chips in a food processor. Process until completely smooth. Stir in the chocolate chips.

Prepare an 8 x 8 pan. You can either rub butter on the bottom inside, or use aluminium foil. This will make removal from the pan easier once the brownies have cooled.

Once the pan is prepared, pour in the mix.

Bake 18 minutes.

Remove from oven and cool completely before cutting. If they still look a bit undercooked, they can be chilled in the fridge overnight to firm up.

Greek Salad

Total time: 40 minutes
Prep time: 10 minutes
Serves: 6

Ingredients

Salad

1 English cucumber, unpeeled, seeded, and sliced 1/4-inch thick
1 orange bell pepper, seeded and large-diced
1 yellow bell pepper, seeded and large-diced

1 pint grape tomatoes, halved
1/2 red onion, sliced in half-rounds
4 oz feta cheese (optional)
1/2 cup black or calamata olives, pitted

Vinaigrette
2 cloves garlic, minced
1 tsp dried oregano
1/2 tsp Dijon mustard
1/4 cup good red wine vinegar
1 tsp kosher salt
1/2 tsp freshly ground black pepper
1/2 cup good olive oil

Directions

Place the cucumber, peppers, tomatoes, and red onion in a large bowl.

In a separate bowl, whisk together the garlic, oregano, mustard, vinegar, salt, and pepper. To emulsify the vinaigrette, slowly add the olive oil while still whisking.

Pour the vinaigrette over the vegetables. Add the feta (if desired) and olives and toss lightly.

Set aside for 30 minutes to allow the flavors to blend. Serve at room temperature.

Liver-Friendly Potato Salad

Total time: 13-18 minutes
Prep time: 3 minutes

Cook time: 10-15 minutes
Serves: 6-8

Ingredients

4 large potatoes, cubed (about 1-inch)
1/2 cup lemon juice
2 tsp mustard powder or turmeric powder
1/2 tsp cumin seeds (optional)
1 1/2 tsp sea salt
1 red small onion, finely chopped
2 cloves garlic, minced
1/2 cup extra virgin olive oil
Your choice of fresh, chopped herbs (2 tbsp of fresh parsley work great!)

Directions

Steam the potatoes until fork tender (about 10-15 minutes).

In a small bowl, mix lemon juice, mustard or turmeric powder, cumin seeds (optional), and salt. Place the steamed potatoes in a large bowl, pour the lemon juice mixture over the potatoes, add the onions and garlic, and stir gently to coat the potatoes. Cover and place in the refrigerator to cool.

When the potatoes are cool, pour olive oil over them, add fresh herbs, and stir well.

Serve chilled or at room temperature.

Grain Free Bircher-Style Muesli

Ingredients

    1 red unpeeled apple, coarsely grated
    1 tsp lime juice
    1 tbsp chia seeds
    2 tbsp chopped pecans
    2 tbsp flaked almonds
    2 tbsp unsweetened shredded coconut
    1 tbsp hemp seeds
    A pinch of cinnamon and clove powder
    ½ cup milk of your choice

Directions

Mix all ingredients together and place in an airtight container. Leave in the fridge overnight.

The next morning, top with fruit of your choice and enjoy.

CHAPTER NINE
HOME REMEDIES FOR FATTY LIVER DISEASE

Rounding out this book are some extra things you can add to your diet that can help you with your fatty liver and your overall healthy lifestyle. There are many websites out there for healthy eating and for things concerning those who have FLD. Generally, they are listed as "liver friendly."

The home remedies listed here are not things you have to do, but they can help you in your journey, especially if you need variety in your life. Adding one of these home remedies to your diet can make you feel like you are on a taste-testing adventure, rather than feeling trapped within your new healthy lifestyle. And they're good for you!

1. Apple Cider Vinegar

This sweet vinegar can help get rid of some of the fat that has accumulated in our bodies, including our liver. It can also promote liver function and reduce liver inflammation.

Add one tablespoon of apple cider vinegar to a glass of warm water and stir. Add honey for additional flavor. Drink once or twice daily, preferably before meals.

2. Lemon

Vitamin C is your friend. It helps the liver produce glutathione, which neutralizes toxins. Many foods high in Vitamin C are listed in this book, but lemons are a great choice. Besides containing Vitamin C, lemons contain naringenin, which may help reduce liver inflammation.

Either squeeze half a lemon in a glass of water or over any food, such as a salad. You can also add fresh-squeezed lemon juice to any fruit and/or vegetable smoothie you make, as well.

3. Dandelion

Dandelion can be great to detoxify your body and reduce the fat in your liver.

Put dandelion root in a cup of warm water and let sit for 10 minutes. Strain the water and add a bit of honey to it for extra flavor.

You can also add some of the leaves to a salad.

You should avoid consuming dandelions if you are pregnant or diabetic.

4. Green Tea

Green tea is healthy for a number of reasons, but most importantly for our purposes here, it contains catechins, which may help improve liver function. It can also reduce fat in the body.

It is good to drink green tea throughout the day, generally about 3 to 4 cups.

5. Turmeric

Turmeric can help the body digest fat easier. The less fat in your body, the less build-up there is.

Mix turmeric powder in a glass of warm water. Drink it one to two times a day.

CHAPTER TEN
FINAL MESSAGE

0As mentioned at the beginning of this book, this is meant to be a helpful guide to those who have Fatty Liver Disease (FLD) who wish to do additional research. While I highly recommend doing your own research, this book gives you a very good starting point, as it should answer many of your questions and give you things to discuss with your doctor.

FLD is very serious, and the fact that we may very well have it and not know about it should make all of us consider living a healthier lifestyle. While there are certainly a lot of things out there that are not healthy for us, we can enjoy them so long as we allow our liver to process the them and help it out with healthy eating and exercise.

If you have FLD, then you need to work to do what you can to undo it. You need to dedicate the rest of your life to living a healthy lifestyle to prevent it from getting worse. Hopefully, if you do develop FLD (which I hope no one does), it is because you are in your 40s and have already lived a life of culinary curiosity, so you can be more focused on maintaining your health as much as possible.

I do stress however that being healthy should start in our youth and continue throughout our lives. Not just to prevent FLD, but to promote lifelong energy and longevity.

Take heed of the advice in this book, whether to overcome or prevent FLD, so you can live a long and happy life.

Printed in Great Britain
by Amazon